STAGE 3 KIDNEY DISEASE DIET COOKBOOK FOR SENIORS

A Complete Guide to Managing Chronic Kidney Disease with Easy, Delicious, and Healthy Recipes for Stage 3 - Low Sodium, Low Potassium, Low Phosphorus, and Meal Plans.

Richie Smile Walker

Copyright © 2024

All Rights Are Reserved

The content in this book may not be reproduced, duplicated, or transferred without the express written permission of the author or publisher. Under no circumstances will the publisher or author be held liable or legally responsible for any losses, expenditures, or damages incurred directly or indirectly as a consequence of the information included in this book.

Legal Remarks

Copyright protection applies to this publication. It is only intended for personal use. No piece of this work may be modified, distributed, sold, quoted, or paraphrased without the author's or publisher's consent.

Disclaimer Statement

Please keep in mind that the contents of this booklet are meant for educational and recreational purposes. Every effort has been made to offer accurate, up-to-date, reliable, and thorough information. There are, however, no stated or implied assurances of any kind. Readers understand that the author is providing competent counsel. The content in this book originates from several sources. Please seek the opinion of a competent professional before using any of the tactics outlined in this book. By reading this book, the reader agrees that the author will not be held accountable for any direct or indirect damages resulting from the use of the information contained therein, including, but not limited to, errors, omissions, or inaccuracies.

TABLE OF CONTENTS

INTRODUCTION

Navigating the complexities of kidney disease, especially in its third stage, can be a daunting task. You're not just managing a condition; you're altering a lifestyle, reshaping habits, and, most importantly, transforming your diet. This cookbook is more than just a collection of recipes; it's a companion on your journey to maintaining kidney health and enhancing your quality of life through the power of nutrition.

Introduction to Stage 3 Kidney Disease

If you or a loved one has been diagnosed with stage 3 kidney disease, you're in a pivotal phase. This stage is a middle ground, a wake-up call that your kidneys are under strain and need your attention and care. The kidneys, those bean-shaped organs that filter waste from your blood and regulate fluid levels, are now working below their normal capacity. You might feel overwhelmed, scared, or even a bit lost. That's perfectly normal.

Stage 3 kidney disease is often detected through a decrease in the glomerular filtration rate (GFR), signaling that your kidneys are not working as efficiently as they should. Symptoms might start to become more noticeable. You could experience fatigue, fluid retention, changes in urination patterns, and other signs that your body isn't quite in harmony. But here's the silver lining: with the right approach, especially through diet, you can play a significant role in managing your condition and slowing its progression.

Understanding the Importance of Diet in Managing Kidney Disease

Diet plays a crucial role in managing kidney disease. The foods you eat can either alleviate or exacerbate your condition. It's all about balance and making informed choices. Certain nutrients, like potassium, phosphorus, sodium, and protein, become particularly important. Too much or too little of these can affect your kidney function and overall well-being.

But it's not just about limiting or avoiding certain foods. It's about embracing a diet that supports your kidneys, nourishes your body, and still delights your taste buds. Yes, you heard that right. A kidney-friendly diet doesn't have to be bland or restrictive. With the right guidance, you can enjoy delicious meals that are both nutritious and supportive of your kidney health.

How This Cookbook Can Help

This is where our journey together begins. This cookbook is designed with you in mind. It's a guide to transforming your diet without sacrificing flavor or joy. Each recipe has been carefully crafted to be kidney-friendly, easy to prepare, and, most importantly, delicious. We've taken the guesswork out of what to eat by providing you with a variety of recipes that cater to different tastes and dietary needs.

But this cookbook is more than just recipes. It's a source of knowledge and empowerment. We'll dive into the specifics of stage 3 kidney disease, helping you understand how your diet impacts your kidney function. We'll explore the nutrients that are vital to your health and teach you how to create balanced meals that support your kidneys.

We understand that change can be challenging, especially when it comes to something as personal and fundamental as your diet. But you're not alone. Think of this cookbook as a friend, one who understands what you're going through and is here to support you every step of the way. We know the importance of enjoying your food, sharing meals with loved ones, and living a life full of flavor and joy. Our goal is to help you do just that, all while taking care of your kidneys.

As you turn these pages, you'll find more than just recipes. You'll discover tips for reading food labels, advice on managing fluid intake, and strategies for dining out without derailing your diet. We've also included tools to help you plan your meals and track your nutritional intake, making it easier to stay on course.

CHAPTER ONE

UNDERSTANDING STAGE 3 KIDNEY DISEASE

What is Stage 3 Kidney Disease?

Stage 3 kidney disease marks a pivotal point in the progression of chronic kidney disease (CKD), characterized by moderate damage to the kidneys. This stage is further subdivided into two: stage 3A (with a glomerular filtration rate, or GFR, of 45-59 ml/min/1.73 m2) and stage 3B (with a GFR of 30-44 ml/min/1.73 m2). The GFR is a crucial measure, indicating how well the kidneys are filtering waste and excess fluid from the blood.

The kidneys play a vital role in the body, not only in filtering waste but also in regulating blood pressure, electrolyte balance, and red blood cell production. When they're damaged, their ability to perform these functions diminishes, leading to the accumulation of harmful levels of fluid and waste in the body. Stage 3 kidney disease signifies that the kidneys are not functioning as well as they should, but not to the extent that requires dialysis or a kidney transplant.

The progression to stage 3 often occurs gradually and can be due to various causes, including diabetes, high blood pressure, and chronic glomerulonephritis. Early detection and management are crucial in slowing the progression of kidney disease, preserving kidney function, and preventing further complications.

Symptoms and Diagnosis

Many individuals with stage 3 kidney disease do not experience symptoms. When symptoms do occur, they may include fatigue, swelling in the hands and feet (edema), back pain, and changes in urination (such as foamy or dark urine). Because these symptoms can be attributed to a variety of conditions, CKD is often discovered through routine blood and urine tests.

Diagnosis involves measuring the GFR, typically calculated from serum creatinine levels in the blood, along with age, sex, and race. A GFR of 30-59 ml/min/1.73 m2 indicates stage 3 CKD. Additional tests may include urine tests for protein (indicating kidney damage), imaging tests to assess kidney structure, and possibly a kidney biopsy to determine the cause of the kidney disease.

How Diet Affects Kidney Health

Diet plays a critical role in managing kidney disease and preserving kidney function, especially in stage 3 CKD. The kidneys are responsible for filtering waste products from the foods we eat, so when they're damaged, modifying one's diet can help reduce the kidneys' workload and prevent further damage.

A diet high in certain nutrients can exacerbate kidney damage. For example, excessive sodium intake can increase blood pressure, worsening kidney damage. Similarly, high intake of potassium and phosphorus can cause dangerous imbalances in patients with reduced kidney function, as the kidneys struggle to maintain proper levels in the blood.

Conversely, a kidney-friendly diet can help manage blood pressure, prevent fluid retention, and reduce the risk of further kidney damage. This involves limiting foods high in sodium, potassium, and phosphorus while ensuring adequate protein intake that's not too high or too low. The right diet can also help manage other CKD risk factors, such as diabetes and heart disease.

Nutritional Guidelines for Managing Kidney Disease

Managing stage 3 kidney disease through diet involves several key nutritional guidelines:

Sodium: Limiting sodium intake to help control blood pressure and reduce fluid retention. This means avoiding processed foods, canned goods, and salty snacks, and instead choosing fresh, whole foods.

Potassium: While potassium is essential for nerve and muscle function, too much can be harmful when your kidneys are not fully functional. Foods high in potassium, such as bananas, oranges, potatoes, and tomatoes, may need to be limited.

Phosphorus: High phosphorus levels can cause bone and cardiovascular issues in CKD patients. Limiting dairy products, nuts, seeds, and cola beverages can help manage phosphorus levels.

Protein: Protein is essential for growth, healing, and health, but excessive protein can increase the kidneys' workload. A moderate intake of high-quality protein is recommended, with guidance from a healthcare provider or dietitian.

Fluids: Fluid intake may need to be adjusted based on your stage of CKD, especially if you experience fluid retention.

CHAPTER TWO

PLANNING YOUR DIET

Creating a Kidney-Friendly Meal Plan

Navigating the complexities of chronic kidney disease (CKD), particularly at stage 3, requires a thoughtful approach to diet and nutrition. A kidney-friendly meal plan is not just about limiting certain foods and nutrients; it's about creating a balanced, nutritious diet that supports kidney function and overall health. This plan involves understanding the roles of various nutrients, managing fluid intake, and making informed choices about the foods you eat.

Key Components of a Kidney-Friendly Meal Plan

1. **Controlled Protein Intake:** Protein is essential for body repair and immune function but managing its intake is crucial in CKD. Too much protein can increase the kidneys' workload, exacerbating kidney damage. A renal dietitian can help determine the right amount of protein for you, focusing on high-quality sources like lean meats, fish, eggs, and plant-based proteins.

2. **Low Sodium:** High sodium intake can lead to high blood pressure, swelling, and heart issues, which can worsen kidney health. Limiting processed foods, choosing fresh

produce, and using herbs and spices for flavoring instead of salt can help manage sodium intake.

3. **Potassium Management:** While potassium is vital for nerve and muscle function, its levels need to be managed in CKD to prevent heart problems. Depending on your kidney function, you may need to limit high-potassium foods like bananas, potatoes, and tomatoes, or choose lower-potassium alternatives.

4. **Phosphorus Control:** Excess phosphorus can lead to bone and cardiovascular issues in CKD patients. Limiting foods high in phosphorus, such as dairy products, nuts, and seeds, is often necessary.

5. **Fluids:** Fluid intake might need adjustment based on your stage of CKD and whether you experience fluid retention. Monitoring and managing fluid intake can help prevent swelling and heart strain.

6. **Calories:** Ensuring adequate caloric intake is important, especially if you're losing weight without trying. Your dietitian can help adjust your meal plan to ensure you're getting enough calories, possibly through healthy fats and carbohydrates.

Implementing Your Meal Plan

- **Meal Timing and Frequency:** Eating regular meals and snacks can help manage energy levels and prevent overeating. Planning your meals and snacks can also ensure you're getting a balanced intake of nutrients throughout the day.

- **Portion Control:** Understanding portion sizes can help manage your intake of key nutrients, especially protein, sodium, and potassium.

- **Food Preparation:** Cooking methods can affect the nutritional content of your meals. For example, boiling vegetables can reduce their potassium content, making them more kidney-friendly.

- **Label Reading:** Becoming proficient in reading food labels can help you make informed choices about packaged foods, especially regarding their sodium, potassium, and phosphorus content.

Essential Vitamins and Minerals

In CKD, managing the intake of certain vitamins and minerals becomes crucial, as the kidneys' ability to balance these nutrients is compromised. It's important to focus on vitamins and minerals that support kidney health, such as B vitamins, vitamin C, vitamin D (for bone health), and iron (to prevent anemia). However, some vitamins and minerals may need to be limited or supplemented, depending on your specific kidney function and nutritional needs.

Foods to Enjoy and Foods to Avoid

Focusing on fresh, whole foods is key in a kidney-friendly diet. Enjoy fruits and vegetables with lower potassium levels, lean proteins, whole grains, and healthy fats. Avoid high-sodium processed foods, high-potassium fruits and vegetables, and dairy products high in phosphorus.

Supplements and Kidney Health

Supplementation may be necessary for some CKD patients, especially for those vitamins and minerals that are difficult to manage through diet alone. However, it's crucial to consult with a healthcare provider before starting any supplements, as some can be harmful to kidney health or interfere with medications.

CHAPTER THREE

DIETARY MANAGEMENT FOR STAGE 3 KIDNEY DISEASE

The Role of Diet in Slowing Kidney Disease Progression

The progression of chronic kidney disease (CKD) can be significantly influenced by dietary choices. A well-planned diet not only helps in managing the symptoms and complications associated with kidney disease but also plays a crucial role in decelerating its progression. The primary goals of a kidney-friendly diet are to reduce the workload on the kidneys, maintain optimal body functions, and prevent the accumulation of harmful substances in the blood.

Key Dietary Strategies:

1. **Protein Intake Management:** Protein is essential for growth, repair, and overall health, but in CKD, the kidneys may struggle to filter the waste products of protein metabolism. Adjusting protein intake to moderate levels can help reduce the kidneys' workload, slowing disease progression. The exact amount of protein recommended can vary based on the stage of CKD, body size, and other health factors.

2. **Control of Blood Pressure:** High blood pressure is both a cause and a consequence of kidney disease. A diet low in sodium and rich in fruits and vegetables can help control blood pressure. The DASH (Dietary Approaches to Stop Hypertension) diet is often recommended for individuals with CKD.

3. **Blood Sugar Management:** Diabetes is a leading cause of CKD. Managing blood sugar levels through a balanced diet can help prevent or delay the progression of kidney disease. This includes limiting simple sugars and refined carbohydrates while emphasizing complex carbohydrates, fiber, and lean protein.

4. **Electrolyte Balance:** The kidneys play a key role in maintaining electrolyte balance. In CKD, potassium, phosphorus, and sodium levels can become unbalanced, leading to various health issues. Managing the intake of these nutrients is crucial.

5. **Fluid Intake Regulation:** As CKD progresses, the kidneys' ability to regulate fluid balance decreases, leading to fluid retention and swelling. Adjusting fluid intake based on the stage of CKD and the presence of symptoms like edema is important.

Nutrients to Watch: Potassium, Phosphorus, Sodium, and Protein

Managing the intake of certain nutrients is critical in CKD to prevent complications and slow disease progression.

- **Potassium:** High levels can lead to dangerous heart rhythms. Low-potassium foods include apples, berries, and rice.

- **Phosphorus:** Excess phosphorus can cause bone and cardiovascular issues. Foods low in phosphorus include egg whites, bread, and many types of rice.

- **Sodium:** High sodium intake can increase blood pressure and swelling. Opt for fresh, unprocessed foods to keep sodium intake in check.

- **Protein:** While essential, it's important to consume just the right amount to avoid overburdening the kidneys.

Fluid Intake: How Much is Too Much?

Fluid management is a balancing act in CKD. Too little fluid can lead to dehydration, while too much can cause hypertension, swelling, and heart issues. The right amount depends on the stage of CKD, urine output, and whether conditions like diabetes are present. Generally, fluid intake is adjusted to match urine output plus any additional losses (like sweating), with adjustments made based on symptoms and lab results.

Reading Food Labels: A Guide for Seniors

Reading food labels is crucial for managing CKD, as it helps in making informed choices about sodium, potassium, phosphorus, and protein content.

- **Sodium:** Look for "low sodium" or "no salt added" labels. Be wary of terms like "sodium-free," which can still contain sodium.

- **Potassium and Phosphorus:** These may not always be listed, so knowing which foods typically contain these minerals can help. Phosphorus additives in processed foods are a hidden source to be aware of.

- **Protein:** Pay attention to serving sizes to accurately gauge protein intake.

BREAKFAST RECIPES

Low-Potassium Apple Cinnamon Oatmeal

Ingredients:

- 1 cup water
- ½ cup rolled oats
- 1 apple, peeled and diced
- ½ teaspoon cinnamon
- 1 tablespoon honey or maple syrup (optional)
- ¼ cup low-fat milk or almond milk

Prep Time: 5 mins

Cooking Time: 10 mins

Total Time: 15 mins

Servings: 2

Nutrition Facts (per serving):

- Calories: 150
- Fat: 2g
- Saturated Fat: 0.5g
- Cholesterol: 2mg
- Sodium: 30mg

- Carbohydrate: 31g

- Protein: 4g

- Phosphorus: 120mg

- Potassium: 200mg

- Fiber: 4g

- Calcium: 60mg

Instructions:

1. Bring water to a boil in a small saucepan. Add oats and diced apple, reducing heat to a simmer.

2. Stir in cinnamon and continue to cook until oats are soft and water is absorbed about 5-7 minutes.

3. Remove from heat and stir in honey or maple syrup if desired. Allow to cool slightly before stirring in milk.

4. Serve warm, sprinkled with additional cinnamon if desired.

Kidney-Friendly Egg Muffins

Ingredients:

- 6 large eggs

- ¼ cup low-fat milk

- ½ cup diced red bell pepper

- ½ cup diced green bell pepper

- ¼ cup shredded low-sodium cheese

- Salt and pepper to taste

Prep Time: 10 mins

Cooking Time: 20 mins

Total Time: 30 mins

Servings: 6

Nutrition Facts (per serving):

- Calories: 100

- Fat: 7g

- Saturated Fat: 3g

- Cholesterol: 185mg

- Sodium: 125mg

- Carbohydrate: 2g

- Protein: 7g

- Phosphorus: 95mg

- Potassium: 150mg

- Fiber: 0.5g

- Calcium: 60mg

Instructions:

1. Preheat oven to 350°F (175°C). Grease a 6-cup muffin tin or line with muffin liners.

2. Whisk together eggs and milk in a bowl. Stir in diced bell peppers and cheese. Season with salt and pepper.

3. Pour the egg mixture evenly into the prepared muffin cups.

4. Bake for 20 minutes, or until muffins are set and lightly golden on top.

5. Let cool for a few minutes before removing from the tin. Serve warm.

Berry Smoothie Bowl

Ingredients:

- 1 cup frozen mixed berries (strawberries, blueberries, raspberries)

- ½ banana, sliced

- ½ cup low-fat Greek yogurt

- ¼ cup almond milk

- 1 tablespoon chia seeds

- 1 tablespoon honey (optional)

Prep Time: 5 mins

Cooking Time: 0 mins

Total Time: 5 mins

Servings: 1

***Nutrition Facts (per serving):**

- Calories: 285

- Fat: 4.5g

- Saturated Fat: 0.5g

- Cholesterol: 10mg

- Sodium: 55mg

- Carbohydrate: 53g

- Protein: 14g

- Phosphorus: 220mg

- Potassium: 450mg

- Fiber: 8g

- Calcium: 150mg

***Instructions:**

1. In a blender, combine frozen berries, banana, Greek yogurt, almond milk, and honey if using. Blend until smooth.

2. Pour the smoothie into a bowl and top with sliced banana, a sprinkle of chia seeds, and additional berries if desired.

3. Serve immediately, enjoying the creamy texture and burst of flavors.

Avocado Toast with Poached Egg

Ingredients:

- 2 slices whole-grain bread

- 1 ripe avocado

- 2 eggs

- Vinegar (for poaching eggs)

- Salt and pepper to taste

- Red pepper flakes (optional)

Prep Time: 5 mins

Cooking Time: 10 mins

Total Time: 15 mins

Servings: 2

Nutrition Facts (per serving):

- Calories: 320

- Fat: 20g

- Saturated Fat: 4g

- Cholesterol: 185mg

- Sodium: 300mg

- Carbohydrate: 27g

- Protein: 13g

- Phosphorus: 200mg

- Potassium: 500mg

- Fiber: 9g

- Calcium: 60mg

Instructions:

1. Toast the bread slices to your liking.

2. Mash the avocado in a bowl and season with salt and pepper. Spread evenly on the toasted bread.

3. Bring a pot of water to a gentle simmer and add a splash of vinegar. Crack an egg into a cup and gently pour it into the simmering water. Repeat with the second egg. Poach for 3-4 minutes or until the whites are set but yolks remain runny.

4. Carefully remove the eggs with a slotted spoon and place them on top of the avocado toast. Season with salt, pepper, and red pepper flakes if desired.

5. Serve immediately, enjoying the creamy avocado and rich, runny yolk.

Quinoa Breakfast Porridge

Ingredients:

- ½ cup quinoa, rinsed

- 1 cup water

- ½ cup low-fat milk or almond milk

- 1 apple, peeled and diced

- ½ teaspoon cinnamon

- 1 tablespoon honey or maple syrup (optional)

- ¼ cup walnuts, chopped (optional)

Prep Time: 5 mins

Cooking Time: 20 mins

Total Time: 25 mins

Servings: 2

Nutrition Facts (per serving):

- Calories: 235

- Fat: 5g

- Saturated Fat: 0.5g

- Cholesterol: 0mg

- Sodium: 30mg

- Carbohydrate: 42g

- Protein: 8g

- Phosphorus: 150mg

- Potassium: 300mg

- Fiber: 5g

- Calcium: 60mg

Instructions:

1. In a small saucepan, bring water to a boil. Add quinoa, reduce heat to low, cover, and simmer for 15 minutes or until water is absorbed.

2. Stir in milk, diced apple, and cinnamon. Cook for an additional 5 minutes, stirring occasionally.

3. Remove from heat and stir in honey or maple syrup if desired. Serve in bowls topped with chopped walnuts if using.

Spinach and Mushroom Egg White Omelette

Ingredients:

- 4 egg whites

- 1 cup fresh spinach, chopped

- ½ cup mushrooms, sliced

- 2 tablespoons low-sodium feta cheese, crumbled

- 1 teaspoon olive oil

- Salt and pepper to taste

Prep Time: 5 mins

Cooking Time: 8 mins

Total Time: 13 mins

Servings: 1

Nutrition Facts (per serving):

- Calories: 150

- Fat: 6g

- Saturated Fat: 2g

- Cholesterol: 10mg

- Sodium: 200mg

- Carbohydrate: 4g

- Protein: 18g

- Phosphorus: 100mg

- Potassium: 300mg

- Fiber: 1g

- Calcium: 150mg

Instructions:

1. Heat olive oil in a non-stick skillet over medium heat.

2. Sauté mushrooms until they begin to brown, about 3-4 minutes. Add spinach and cook until wilted, about 1-2 minutes.

3. In a bowl, whisk together egg whites, salt, and pepper. Pour over the vegetables in the skillet.

4. Cook until the egg whites are set, about 2-3 minutes. Sprinkle feta cheese over half of the omelette.

5.   Fold the omelet in half and serve hot.

Banana Walnut Pancakes

Ingredients:

- 1 cup whole wheat flour

- 1 tablespoon sugar

- 2 teaspoons baking powder (low sodium)

- 1 cup low-fat milk

- 2 egg whites

- 1 ripe banana, mashed

- ¼ cup walnuts, chopped

- Cooking spray

Prep Time: 10 mins

Cooking Time: 10 mins

Total Time: 20 mins

Servings: 4

Nutrition Facts (per serving):

- Calories: 210

- Fat: 5g

- Saturated Fat: 0.5g

- Cholesterol: 0mg

- Sodium: 75mg

- Carbohydrate: 35g

- Protein: 8g

- Phosphorus: 150mg

- Potassium: 250mg

- Fiber: 4g

- Calcium: 100mg

Instructions:

1. In a large bowl, mix flour, sugar, and baking powder.

2. In another bowl, whisk together milk and egg whites. Stir in mashed banana.

3. Add the wet ingredients to the dry ingredients, stirring until just combined. Fold in chopped walnuts.

4. Heat a non-stick skillet over medium heat and lightly coat with cooking spray.

5. Pour ¼ cup of batter for each pancake and cook until bubbles form on the surface, then flip and cook until golden brown.

6. Serve warm.

Pear and Cottage Cheese Toast

Ingredients:

- 2 slices whole-grain bread

- ½ cup low-fat cottage cheese

- 1 pear, thinly sliced

- 1 teaspoon honey

- Cinnamon to taste

Prep Time: 5 mins

Cooking Time: 2 mins

Total Time: 7 mins

Servings: 2

Nutrition Facts (per serving):

- Calories: 200

- Fat: 2g

- Saturated Fat: 0.5g

- Cholesterol: 5mg

- Sodium: 200mg

- Carbohydrate: 35g

- Protein: 12g

- Phosphorus: 100mg

- Potassium: 200mg

- Fiber: 5g

- Calcium: 80mg

Instructions:

1. Toast the bread slices to your preference.

2. Spread cottage cheese evenly over each slice of toast.

3. Arrange pear slices on top of the cottage cheese.

4. Drizzle with honey and sprinkle with cinnamon before serving.

Zucchini and Bell Pepper Frittata

Ingredients:

- 4 egg whites

- 2 whole eggs

- 1 zucchini, thinly sliced

- 1 red bell pepper, diced

- ¼ cup low-fat milk

- ¼ cup low-sodium shredded cheese

- 1 tablespoon olive oil

- Salt and pepper to taste

Prep Time: 10 mins

Cooking Time: 15 mins

Total Time: 25 mins

Servings: 4

Nutrition Facts (per serving):

- Calories: 150

- Fat: 8g

- Saturated Fat: 2g

- Cholesterol: 105mg

- Sodium: 170mg

- Carbohydrate: 6g

- Protein: 12g

- Phosphorus: 125mg

- Potassium: 250mg

- Fiber: 1g

- Calcium: 100mg

Instructions:

1. Preheat oven to 375°F (190°C).

2. Heat olive oil in an oven-safe skillet over medium heat. Add zucchini and bell pepper, sautéing until tender.

3. In a bowl, whisk together egg whites, whole eggs, milk, salt, and pepper. Pour over the vegetables in the skillet.

4. Sprinkle shredded cheese on top and transfer the skillet to the oven.

5. Bake until the frittata is set and lightly golden, about 12-15 minutes.

6. Cut into wedges and serve hot.

Almond Butter and Blueberry Smoothie

Ingredients:

- 1 cup unsweetened almond milk

- ½ banana

- ½ cup blueberries (fresh or frozen)

- 2 tablespoons almond butter

- 1 tablespoon flaxseed meal

Prep Time: 5 mins

Cooking Time: 0 mins

Total Time: 5 mins

Servings: 1

Nutrition Facts (per serving):

- Calories: 280

- Fat: 15g

- Saturated Fat: 1.5g

- Cholesterol: 0mg

- Sodium: 180mg

- Carbohydrate: 30g

- Protein: 8g

- Phosphorus: 200mg

- Potassium: 400mg

- Fiber: 7g

- Calcium: 300mg

Instructions:

1. In a blender, combine almond milk, banana, blueberries, almond butter, and flaxseed meal.

2. Blend until smooth and creamy.

3. Pour into a glass and serve immediately, enjoying the creamy texture and rich, nutty flavor paired with the sweetness of blueberries.

LUNCH RECIPES

Tuna and White Bean Salad

Ingredients:

- 1 can (15 ounces) low-sodium white beans, rinsed and drained
- 1 can (5 ounces) low-sodium tuna, drained and flaked
- 1 small red onion, finely chopped
- 1 red bell pepper, diced
- 2 tablespoons olive oil
- 1 tablespoon lemon juice
- 1 teaspoon dried oregano
- Salt and pepper to taste
- Fresh parsley, chopped (for garnish)

Prep Time: 10 mins

Cooking Time: 0 mins

Total Time: 10 mins

Servings: 4

Nutrition Facts (per serving):

- Calories: 220

- Fat: 7g

- Saturated Fat: 1g

- Cholesterol: 30mg

- Sodium: 180mg

- Carbohydrate: 22g

- Protein: 20g

- Phosphorus: 150mg

- Potassium: 400mg

- Fiber: 6g

- Calcium: 80mg

Instructions:

1. In a large bowl, combine white beans, tuna, red onion, and red bell pepper.

2. In a small bowl, whisk together olive oil, lemon juice, oregano, salt, and pepper.

3. Pour the dressing over the tuna and bean mixture. Toss gently to combine.

4. Garnish with fresh parsley before serving. Enjoy this refreshing salad as a light and nutritious lunch option.

Chicken and Avocado Wrap

Ingredients:

- 2 whole-grain tortillas

- 1 cup cooked chicken breast, shredded

- 1 ripe avocado, sliced

- ½ cup shredded lettuce

- ¼ cup diced tomatoes

- 2 tablespoons low-fat Greek yogurt

- Salt and pepper to taste

Prep Time: 15 mins

Cooking Time: 0 mins

Total Time: 15 mins

Servings: 2

Nutrition Facts (per serving):

- Calories: 350

- Fat: 15g

- Saturated Fat: 3g

- Cholesterol: 60mg

- Sodium: 300mg

- Carbohydrate: 30g

- Protein: 25g

- Phosphorus: 200mg

- Potassium: 500mg

- Fiber: 7g

- Calcium: 100mg

Instructions:

1. Lay out the tortillas on a flat surface. Spread Greek yogurt evenly across each tortilla.

2. Divide the shredded chicken, avocado slices, shredded lettuce, and diced tomatoes between the two tortillas.

3. Season with salt and pepper to taste.

4. Carefully roll up the tortillas, folding in the sides to hold the filling.

5. Cut each wrap in half and serve immediately for a satisfying and kidney-friendly lunch.

Quinoa Veggie Salad

Ingredients:

- 1 cup cooked quinoa

- ½ cup cherry tomatoes, halved

- ½ cucumber, diced

- ¼ cup red bell pepper, diced

- ¼ cup carrot, shredded

- 2 tablespoons chopped fresh parsley

- 2 tablespoons lemon juice

- 1 tablespoon olive oil

- Salt and pepper to taste

Prep Time: 10 mins

Cooking Time: 0 mins (assuming quinoa is pre-cooked)

Total Time: 10 mins

Servings: 2

Nutrition Facts (per serving):

- Calories: 250

- Fat: 8g

- Saturated Fat: 1g

- Cholesterol: 0mg

- Sodium: 30mg

- Carbohydrate: 38g

- Protein: 8g

- Phosphorus: 150mg

- Potassium: 450mg

- Fiber: 5g

- Calcium: 40mg

Instructions:

1. In a large bowl, combine the cooked quinoa, cherry tomatoes, cucumber, red bell pepper, carrot, and parsley.

2. In a small bowl, whisk together lemon juice, olive oil, salt, and pepper.

3. Pour the dressing over the quinoa mixture and toss to combine.

4. Serve the salad chilled or at room temperature for a light and nutritious lunch.

Broccoli and Almond Soup

Ingredients:

- 2 cups broccoli florets

- 1 small onion, chopped

- 2 cloves garlic, minced

- 4 cups low-sodium vegetable broth

- ¼ cup almonds, toasted and chopped

- 1 tablespoon olive oil

- Salt and pepper to taste

Prep Time: 10 mins

Cooking Time: 20 mins

Total Time: 30 mins

Servings: 4

Nutrition Facts (per serving):

- Calories: 120

- Fat: 7g

- Saturated Fat: 1g

- Cholesterol: 0mg

- Sodium: 150mg

- Carbohydrate: 12g

- Protein: 5g

- Phosphorus: 100mg

- Potassium: 300mg

- Fiber: 3g

- Calcium: 50mg

Instructions:

1. Heat olive oil in a large pot over medium heat. Add onion and garlic, sautéing until softened.

2. Add broccoli and vegetable broth. Bring to a boil, then reduce heat and simmer until broccoli is tender, about 15 minutes.

3. Use an immersion blender to puree the soup until smooth. Season with salt and pepper to taste.

4. Serve the soup garnished with toasted almonds for a comforting and kidney-friendly meal.

Mediterranean Lentil Salad

Ingredients:

- 1 cup cooked lentils

- ½ cup diced cucumber

- ½ cup diced tomatoes

- ¼ cup diced red onion

- ¼ cup crumbled feta cheese (low-sodium)

- 2 tablespoons chopped fresh parsley

- 2 tablespoons lemon juice

- 1 tablespoon olive oil

- Salt and pepper to taste

Prep Time: 15 mins

Cooking Time: 0 mins (assuming lentils are pre-cooked)

Total Time: 15 mins

Servings: 2

Nutrition Facts (per serving):

- Calories: 280

- Fat: 10g

- Saturated Fat: 3g

- Cholesterol: 15mg

- Sodium: 200mg

- Carbohydrate: 34g

- Protein: 14g

- Phosphorus: 200mg

- Potassium: 450mg

- Fiber: 8g

- Calcium: 120mg

Instructions:

1. In a large bowl, combine the cooked lentils, cucumber, tomatoes, red onion, and feta cheese.

2. In a small bowl, whisk together lemon juice, olive oil, salt, and pepper.

3. Pour the dressing over the lentil mixture and toss to combine.

4. Garnish with fresh parsley before serving. Enjoy this flavourful and nutritious salad as a perfect lunch for kidney health.

Carrot and Ginger Soup

Ingredients:

- 2 tablespoons olive oil

- 1 onion, chopped

- 2 cloves garlic, minced

- 2 tablespoons grated fresh ginger

- 4 cups chopped carrots

- 4 cups low-sodium vegetable broth

- Salt and pepper to taste

- Fresh parsley, for garnish

Prep Time: 10 mins

Cooking Time: 25 mins

Total Time: 35 mins

Servings: 4

Nutrition Facts (per serving):

- Calories: 150

- Fat: 7g

- Saturated Fat: 1g

- Cholesterol: 0mg

- Sodium: 300mg

- Carbohydrate: 21g

- Protein: 3g

- Phosphorus: 70mg

- Potassium: 470mg

- Fiber: 5g

- Calcium: 40mg

Instructions:

1. Heat olive oil in a large pot over medium heat. Add onion and garlic, and cook until softened.

2. Stir in ginger and carrots, cooking for a few more minutes.

3. Add vegetable broth and bring to a boil. Reduce heat to simmer and cover, cooking until carrots are tender, about 20 minutes.

4. Puree the soup using an immersion blender until smooth. Season with salt and pepper to taste.

5. Serve hot, garnished with fresh parsley.

Roasted Vegetable Quiche

Ingredients:

- 1 pre-made whole-grain pie crust

- 1 cup roasted vegetables (zucchini, bell pepper, and onion)

- 4 eggs

- 1 cup low-fat milk

- ½ cup shredded low-sodium cheese

- Salt and pepper to taste

- 1 tablespoon olive oil (for roasting vegetables)

Prep Time: 15 mins (plus roasting time)

Cooking Time: 35 mins

Total Time: 50 mins

Servings: 6

Nutrition Facts (per serving):

- Calories: 220

- Fat: 12g

- Saturated Fat: 4g

- Cholesterol: 140mg

- Sodium: 200mg

- Carbohydrate: 18g

- Protein: 10g

- Phosphorus: 150mg

- Potassium: 250mg

- Fiber: 2g

- Calcium: 150mg

Instructions:

1. Preheat oven to 375°F (190°C). Toss vegetables with olive oil, salt, and pepper, and roast until tender.

2. Whisk together eggs, milk, salt, and pepper.

3. Spread roasted vegetables evenly over the pie crust. Pour the egg mixture over the vegetables. Sprinkle with cheese.

4. Bake for 35 minutes, or until the quiche is set and the crust is golden brown.

5. Let cool slightly before serving.

Grilled Chicken Caesar Salad

Ingredients:

- 2 boneless, skinless chicken breasts

- 4 cups chopped romaine lettuce

- ¼ cup low-fat Caesar dressing

- 2 tablespoons grated Parmesan cheese (low-sodium)

- 1 cup whole-grain croutons

- Salt and pepper to taste

- 1 tablespoon olive oil (for grilling)

Prep Time: 10 mins

Cooking Time: 15 mins

Total Time: 25 mins

Servings: 2

Nutrition Facts (per serving):

- Calories: 350

- Fat: 15g

- Saturated Fat: 3g

- Cholesterol: 80mg

- Sodium: 400mg

- Carbohydrate: 22g

- Protein: 32g

- Phosphorus: 250mg

- Potassium: 500mg

- Fiber: 3g

- Calcium: 150mg

Instructions:

1. Preheat the grill to medium-high heat. Season chicken breasts with salt and pepper, then brush with olive oil.

2. Grill chicken for 7-8 minutes per side, or until fully cooked. Let rest, then slice thinly.

3. In a large bowl, toss romaine lettuce with Caesar dressing, Parmesan cheese, and croutons.

4. Divide salad among plates, top with grilled chicken slices, and serve immediately.

Baked Salmon with Dill Yogurt Sauce

Ingredients:

- 2 salmon fillets (4 ounces each)

- 1 tablespoon olive oil

- Salt and pepper to taste

- ½ cup low-fat Greek yogurt

- 1 tablespoon chopped fresh dill

- 1 teaspoon lemon juice

- Lemon slices, for garnish

Prep Time: 5 mins

Cooking Time: 15 mins

Total Time: 20 mins

Servings: 2

Nutrition Facts (per serving):

- Calories: 300

- Fat: 18g

- Saturated Fat: 3g

- Cholesterol: 75mg

- Sodium: 200mg

- Carbohydrate: 3g

- Protein: 29g

- Phosphorus: 300mg

- Potassium: 700mg

- Fiber: 0g

- Calcium: 60mg

Instructions:

1. Preheat oven to 375°F (190°C). Place salmon fillets on a baking sheet, drizzle with olive oil, and season with salt and pepper.

2. Bake for 12-15 minutes or until salmon flakes easily with a fork.

3. While salmon is baking, mix Greek yogurt, dill, and lemon juice in a small bowl.

4. Serve salmon with a dollop of dill yogurt sauce and garnish with lemon slices.

Turkey and Cranberry Sandwich

Ingredients:

- 2 slices whole-grain bread

- 4 ounces sliced turkey breast (low-sodium)

- 2 tablespoons cranberry sauce

- 1 tablespoon low-fat cream cheese

- Lettuce leaves

- Salt and pepper to taste

Prep Time: 5 mins

Cooking Time: 0 mins

Total Time: 5 mins

Servings: 1

Nutrition Facts (per serving):

- Calories: 320

- Fat: 4g

- Saturated Fat: 1g

- Cholesterol: 50mg

- Sodium: 300mg

- Carbohydrate: 44g

- Protein: 28g

- Phosphorus: 200mg

- Potassium: 400mg

- Fiber: 6g

- Calcium: 80mg

Instructions:

1. Spread cranberry sauce on one slice of bread and cream cheese on the other.

2. Layer turkey slices and lettuce on one slice of bread, season with salt and pepper, then top with the other slice.

3. Cut the sandwich in half and serve immediately for a refreshing and nutritious lunch option

DINNER RECIPES

Lemon Herb Baked Cod

Ingredients:

- 4 cod fillets (4 ounces each)
- 2 tablespoons olive oil
- 1 lemon, juiced and zested
- 2 cloves garlic, minced
- 1 teaspoon dried thyme
- 1 teaspoon dried parsley
- Salt and pepper to taste
- Lemon slices for garnish

Prep Time: 10 mins

Cooking Time: 15 mins

Total Time: 25 mins

Servings: 4

Nutrition Facts (per serving):

- Calories: 190
- Fat: 7g
- Saturated Fat: 1g

- Cholesterol: 60mg

- Sodium: 150mg

- Carbohydrate: 2g

- Protein: 30g

- Phosphorus: 250mg

- Potassium: 500mg

- Fiber: 0.5g

- Calcium: 30mg

Instructions:

1. Preheat oven to 400°F (200°C). Line a baking sheet with parchment paper.

2. In a small bowl, mix olive oil, lemon juice and zest, garlic, thyme, parsley, salt, and pepper.

3. Place cod fillets on the prepared baking sheet. Brush each fillet with the lemon herb mixture.

4. Bake for 12-15 minutes or until the fish flakes easily with a fork.

5. Serve garnished with lemon slices and a sprinkle of fresh parsley if desired.

Vegetable Stir-Fry with Tofu

Ingredients:

- 1 block (14 ounces) of firm tofu, pressed and cubed

- 2 tablespoons peanut or canola oil, divided

- 2 cups broccoli florets

- 1 red bell pepper, sliced

- 1 carrot, julienned

- 2 tablespoons low-sodium soy sauce

- 1 tablespoon sesame oil

- 1 teaspoon grated fresh ginger

- 2 cloves garlic, minced

- Sesame seeds for garnish

Prep Time: 15 mins

Cooking Time: 10 mins

Total Time: 25 mins

Servings: 4

Nutrition Facts (per serving):

- Calories: 220

- Fat: 14g

- Saturated Fat: 2g

- Cholesterol: 0mg

- Sodium: 300mg

- Carbohydrate: 12g

- Protein: 12g

- Phosphorus: 150mg

- Potassium: 400mg

- Fiber: 3g

- Calcium: 150mg

Instructions:

1. Heat 1 tablespoon oil in a large skillet or wok over medium-high heat. Add tofu cubes and cook until golden brown on all sides. Remove tofu from the skillet and set aside.

2. In the same skillet, add the remaining oil. Sauté broccoli, bell pepper, and carrot until tender-crisp.

3. Add the tofu back to the skillet. Stir in soy sauce, sesame oil, ginger, and garlic. Cook for another 2-3 minutes, stirring frequently.

4. Serve hot, garnished with sesame seeds.

Quinoa Stuffed Bell Peppers

Ingredients:

- 4 large bell peppers, halved and seeded

- 1 cup quinoa, cooked

- 1 can (15 ounces) low-sodium black beans, rinsed and drained

- 1 cup corn kernels (fresh or frozen)

- 1 teaspoon cumin

- 1 teaspoon paprika

- ½ cup low-sodium tomato sauce

- ¼ cup shredded low-sodium cheese (optional)

- 2 tablespoons fresh cilantro, chopped

Prep Time: 20 mins

Cooking Time: 25 mins

Total Time: 45 mins

Servings: 4

Nutrition Facts (per serving):

- Calories: 280

- Fat: 4g

- Saturated Fat: 1g

- Cholesterol: 5mg

- Sodium: 200mg

- Carbohydrate: 50g

- Protein: 14g

- Phosphorus: 200mg

- Potassium: 600mg

- Fiber: 10g

- Calcium: 100mg

Instructions:

1. Preheat oven to 375°F (190°C). Place bell pepper halves in a baking dish, cut side up.

2. In a bowl, mix cooked quinoa, black beans, corn, cumin, paprika, and tomato sauce.

3. Spoon the quinoa mixture into each bell pepper half. Top with shredded cheese if using.

4. Cover with foil and bake for 20 minutes. Uncover and bake for an additional 5 minutes, or until the peppers are tender and the cheese is melted.

5. Garnish with fresh cilantro before serving.

Baked Garlic Parmesan Chicken

Ingredients:

- 4 boneless, skinless chicken breasts

- 2 tablespoons olive oil

- 2 cloves garlic, minced

- ½ cup grated Parmesan cheese (low-sodium)

- 1 teaspoon dried oregano

- 1 teaspoon dried basil

- Salt and pepper to taste

Prep Time: 10 mins

Cooking Time: 20 mins

Total Time: 30 mins

Servings: 4

Nutrition Facts (per serving):

- Calories: 280

- Fat: 14g

- Saturated Fat: 3g

- Cholesterol: 75mg

- Sodium: 250mg

- Carbohydrate: 2g

- Protein: 34g

- Phosphorus: 300mg

- Potassium: 450mg

- Fiber: 0g

- Calcium: 150mg

Instructions:

1. Preheat oven to 400°F (200°C). Line a baking sheet with parchment paper.

2. In a small bowl, mix olive oil, garlic, Parmesan cheese, oregano, basil, salt, and pepper.

3. Place chicken breasts on the prepared baking sheet. Spread the Parmesan mixture evenly over each breast.

4. Bake for 20 minutes, or until chicken is cooked through and the topping is golden.

5. Serve hot, garnished with additional fresh herbs if desired.

Spinach and Feta Stuffed Salmon

Ingredients:

- 4 salmon fillets (4 ounces each)

- 2 cups fresh spinach, chopped

- ½ cup crumbled feta cheese (low-sodium)

- 2 tablespoons olive oil

- Salt and pepper to taste

- Lemon slices for garnish

Prep Time: 15 mins

Cooking Time: 20 mins

Total Time: 35 mins

Servings: 4

Nutrition Facts (per serving):

- Calories: 300

- Fat: 18g

- Saturated Fat: 4g

- Cholesterol: 75mg

- Sodium: 200mg

- Carbohydrate: 2g

- Protein: 30g

- Phosphorus: 350mg

- Potassium: 550mg

- Fiber: 1g

- Calcium: 100mg

Instructions:

1. Preheat oven to 375°F (190°C). Line a baking sheet with parchment paper.

2. In a skillet over medium heat, warm 1 tablespoon olive oil. Add spinach and cook until wilted, about 2-3 minutes. Remove from heat and let cool slightly. Stir in feta cheese.

3. Cut a slit in each salmon fillet to create a pocket. Be careful not to cut all the way through.

4. Stuff each salmon fillet with the spinach and feta mixture. Secure with toothpicks if necessary.

5. Place the stuffed salmon fillets on the prepared baking sheet. Drizzle with the remaining olive oil and season with salt and pepper.

6. Bake for 15-20 minutes, or until salmon is cooked through and flakes easily with a fork.

7. Serve immediately, garnished with lemon slices.

Herb-Roasted Turkey Breast

Ingredients:

- 2 lbs turkey breast

- 2 tablespoons olive oil

- 1 teaspoon dried rosemary

- 1 teaspoon dried thyme

- 1 teaspoon dried sage

- Salt and pepper to taste

- 2 cloves garlic, minced

Prep Time: 10 mins

Cooking Time: 60 mins

Total Time: 70 mins

Servings: 6

Nutrition Facts (per serving):

- Calories: 190

- Fat: 4g

- Saturated Fat: 0.5g

- Cholesterol: 90mg

- Sodium: 75mg

- Carbohydrate: 0g

- Protein: 35g

- Phosphorus: 220mg

- Potassium: 400mg

- Fiber: 0g

- Calcium: 20mg

Instructions:

1. Preheat oven to 325°F (165°C). Place the turkey breast in a roasting pan.

2. In a small bowl, mix olive oil, rosemary, thyme, sage, salt, pepper, and garlic. Rub this mixture all over the turkey breast.

3. Roast in the preheated oven for about 1 hour, or until the internal temperature reaches 165°F (74°C).

4. Let the turkey rest for 10 minutes before slicing. Serve warm.

Cauliflower Rice Stir-Fry

Ingredients:

- 1 head cauliflower, grated into rice-sized pieces

- 2 tablespoons sesame oil

- 1 cup mixed vegetables (carrots, peas, and corn)

- 2 cloves garlic, minced

- 2 tablespoons low-sodium soy sauce

- 1 egg, beaten

- Green onions, sliced for garnish

Prep Time: 15 mins

Cooking Time: 10 mins

Total Time: 25 mins

Servings: 4

Nutrition Facts (per serving):

- Calories: 150

- Fat: 7g

- Saturated Fat: 1g

- Cholesterol: 47mg

- Sodium: 300mg

- Carbohydrate: 15g

- Protein: 7g

- Phosphorus: 120mg

- Potassium: 450mg

- Fiber: 4g

- Calcium: 40mg

Instructions:

1. Heat 1 tablespoon sesame oil in a large skillet over medium heat. Add the minced garlic and sauté until fragrant.

2. Add the mixed vegetables and cook until they are tender.

3. Stir in the grated cauliflower and soy sauce. Cook, stirring frequently, for about 5 minutes.

4. Push the cauliflower rice mixture to the side of the skillet. Add the remaining sesame oil and the beaten egg to the empty side of the skillet. Scramble the egg, then mix it into the cauliflower rice.

5. Serve hot, garnished with green onions.

Grilled Vegetable Platter

Ingredients:

- 1 zucchini, sliced

- 1 yellow squash, sliced

- 1 red bell pepper, cut into strips

- 1 eggplant, sliced

- 2 tablespoons olive oil

- Salt and pepper to taste

- 1 teaspoon dried oregano

Prep Time: 10 mins

Cooking Time: 15 mins

Total Time: 25 mins

Servings: 4

Nutrition Facts (per serving):

- Calories: 120

- Fat: 7g

- Saturated Fat: 1g

- Cholesterol: 0mg

- Sodium: 75mg

- Carbohydrate: 13g

- Protein: 3g

- Phosphorus: 60mg

- Potassium: 450mg

- Fiber: 5g

- Calcium: 30mg

Instructions:

1. Preheat the grill to medium-high heat.

2. Toss the sliced vegetables with olive oil, salt, pepper, and oregano until evenly coated.

3. Grill the vegetables in batches, turning occasionally, until they are tender and have grill marks, about 3-4 minutes per side.

4. Serve the grilled vegetables as a colorful and healthy side dish.

Lemon Dill Salmon Pasta

Ingredients:

- 8 oz whole-grain spaghetti

- 2 salmon fillets (4 ounces each)

- 1 tablespoon olive oil

- Juice and zest of 1 lemon

- 2 tablespoons fresh dill, chopped

- Salt and pepper to taste

- 1 cup low-sodium vegetable broth

Prep Time: 10 mins

Cooking Time: 20 mins

Total Time: 30 mins

Servings: 4

Nutrition Facts (per serving):

- Calories: 320

- Fat: 9g

- Saturated Fat: 1.5g

- Cholesterol: 50mg

- Sodium: 100mg

- Carbohydrate: 40g

- Protein: 22g

- Phosphorus: 250mg

- Potassium: 500mg

- Fiber: 6g

- Calcium: 30mg

Instructions:

1. Cook the spaghetti according to package instructions. Drain and set aside.

2. Heat olive oil in a skillet over medium heat. Season the salmon with salt and pepper, and cook until golden and

flaky, about 4-5 minutes per side. Remove from the skillet and set aside.

3. In the same skillet, add lemon juice, zest, dill, and vegetable broth. Bring to a simmer.

4. Flake the salmon in the skillet with the lemon dill sauce. Toss to combine.

5. Serve the salmon and sauce over the cooked spaghetti.

Balsamic Glazed Chicken

Ingredients:

- 4 boneless, skinless chicken breasts

- 2 tablespoons olive oil

- Salt and pepper to taste

- 1/4 cup balsamic vinegar

- 1 tablespoon honey

- 1 clove garlic, minced

- 1 teaspoon dried thyme

Prep Time: 5 mins

Cooking Time: 20 mins

Total Time: 25 mins

Servings: 4

Nutrition Facts (per serving):

- Calories: 220

- Fat: 8g

- Saturated Fat: 1g

- Cholesterol: 65mg

- Sodium: 200mg

- Carbohydrate: 9g

- Protein: 29g

- Phosphorus: 220mg

- Potassium: 300mg

- Fiber: 0g

- Calcium: 20mg

Instructions:

1. Season chicken breasts with salt and pepper.

2. Heat olive oil in a skillet over medium-high heat. Add chicken and cook until golden and cooked through, about 6-7 minutes per side. Remove chicken from skillet and set aside.

3. In the same skillet, add balsamic vinegar, honey, garlic, and thyme. Stir to combine and bring to a simmer. Cook until the sauce has thickened slightly, about 3-4 minutes. 4. Return the chicken to the skillet, spooning the balsamic glaze over the chicken to coat thoroughly.

5. Cook for an additional 2 minutes, ensuring the chicken is well coated and heated through.

6. Serve the chicken drizzled with any remaining glaze from the skillet.

SNACKS AND DESSERTS

Apple Cinnamon Chips

Ingredients:

- 2 large apples, thinly sliced

- 1 teaspoon ground cinnamon

- Cooking spray

Prep Time: 10 mins

Cooking Time: 2 hours

Total Time: 2 hours 10 mins

Servings: 4

Nutrition Facts (per serving):

- Calories: 50

- Fat: 0g

- Saturated Fat: 0g

- Cholesterol: 0mg

- Sodium: 0mg

- Carbohydrate: 13g

- Protein: 0g

- Phosphorus: 10mg

- Potassium: 100mg

- Fiber: 2g

- Calcium: 10mg

Instructions:

1. Preheat oven to 200°F (93°C). Line two baking sheets with parchment paper and lightly spray with cooking spray.

2. Arrange apple slices in a single layer on the baking sheets. Sprinkle cinnamon evenly over apple slices.

3. Bake for 1 hour, then flip the apple slices and continue baking for another hour, or until the apple slices are dried out but still pliable.

4. Let cool completely on the baking sheets. Serve as a crunchy, sweet snack.

Kidney-Friendly Rice Pudding

Ingredients:

- ½ cup uncooked white rice

- 2 cups water

- 2 cups low-fat milk

- ¼ cup sugar

- 1 teaspoon vanilla extract

- Ground cinnamon for garnish

Prep Time: 5 mins

Cooking Time: 45 mins

Total Time: 50 mins

Servings: 4

Nutrition Facts (per serving):

- Calories: 200

- Fat: 2g

- Saturated Fat: 1g

- Cholesterol: 10mg

- Sodium: 50mg

- Carbohydrate: 40g

- Protein: 6g

- Phosphorus: 100mg

- Potassium: 150mg

- Fiber: 0g

- Calcium: 150mg

Instructions:

1. In a large saucepan, bring water to a boil. Add rice and reduce heat to low. Cover and simmer for 20 minutes, or until water is absorbed.

2. Add milk and sugar to the cooked rice. Cook over medium heat, stirring frequently, until the mixture thickens, about 25 minutes.

3. Remove from heat and stir in vanilla extract.

4. Serve warm or chilled, garnished with a sprinkle of cinnamon.

No-Bake Peanut Butter Balls

Ingredients:

- 1 cup oats

- ½ cup natural peanut butter

- ¼ cup honey

- 1 teaspoon vanilla extract

- 2 tablespoons ground flaxseed

Prep Time: 15 mins

Cooking Time: 0 mins

Total Time: 15 mins (plus chilling time)

Servings: 8

Nutrition Facts (per serving):

- Calories: 180

- Fat: 9g

- Saturated Fat: 2g

- Cholesterol: 0mg

- Sodium: 75mg

- Carbohydrate: 22g

- Protein: 6g

- Phosphorus: 120mg

- Potassium: 150mg

- Fiber: 3g

- Calcium: 20mg

Instructions:

1. In a medium bowl, mix oats, peanut butter, honey, vanilla extract, and ground flaxseed until well combined.

2. Roll the mixture into 1-inch balls and place on a baking sheet lined with parchment paper.

3. Chill in the refrigerator for at least 1 hour before serving. Store in an airtight container in the refrigerator.

Chilled Melon Soup

Ingredients:

- 4 cups cubed melon (cantaloupe or honeydew)

- 1 cup low-fat plain yogurt

- 2 tablespoons honey

- 1 tablespoon fresh lime juice

- Mint leaves for garnish

Prep Time: 10 mins

Cooking Time: 0 mins

Total Time: 10 mins (plus chilling time)

Servings: 4

Nutrition Facts (per serving):

- Calories: 120

- Fat: 1g

- Saturated Fat: 0.5g

- Cholesterol: 5mg

- Sodium: 45mg

- Carbohydrate: 25g

- Protein: 4g

- Phosphorus: 95mg

- Potassium: 400mg

- Fiber: 1g

- Calcium: 120mg

Instructions:

1. In a blender, combine melon, yogurt, honey, and lime juice. Blend until smooth.

2. Chill the soup in the refrigerator for at least 2 hours.

3. Serve cold, garnished with mint leaves.

Baked Pear with Honey and Walnuts

Ingredients:

- 2 pears, halved and cored

- 2 tablespoons honey

- ¼ cup chopped walnuts

- Ground cinnamon for sprinkling

Prep Time: 5 mins

Cooking Time: 25 mins

Total Time: 30 mins

Servings: 4

Nutrition Facts (per serving):

- Calories: 150

- Fat: 5g

- Saturated Fat: 0.5g

- Cholesterol: 0mg

- Sodium: 0mg

- Carbohydrate: 27g

- Protein: 2g

- Phosphorus: 50mg

- Potassium: 175mg

- Fiber: 4g

- Calcium: 20mg

Instructions:

1. Preheat oven to 350°F (175°C). Arrange pear halves cut side up in a baking dish.

2. Drizzle honey over the pears and sprinkle with chopped walnuts and cinnamon.

3. Bake in the preheated oven for 25 minutes, or until pears are tender.

4. Serve warm, with a dollop of low-fat yogurt if desired.

Avocado Chocolate Mousse

Ingredients:

- 2 ripe avocados, peeled and pitted

- 1/4 cup unsweetened cocoa powder

- 1/4 cup honey or maple syrup

- 1/2 teaspoon vanilla extract

- A pinch of salt

- Fresh berries for garnish

Prep Time: 10 mins

Cooking Time: 0 mins

Total Time: 10 mins

Servings: 4

Nutrition Facts (per serving):

- Calories: 240

- Fat: 15g

- Saturated Fat: 2g

- Cholesterol: 0mg

- Sodium: 75mg

- Carbohydrate: 28g

- Protein: 3g

- Phosphorus: 60mg

- Potassium: 487mg

- Fiber: 7g

- Calcium: 20mg

Instructions:

1. In a blender or food processor, combine avocados, cocoa powder, honey or maple syrup, vanilla extract, and a pinch of salt. Blend until smooth and creamy.

2. Divide the mousse into serving dishes and refrigerate for at least 1 hour to set.

3. Serve chilled, garnished with fresh berries.

Cucumber Mint Water

Ingredients:

- 1 large cucumber, thinly sliced

- 10 fresh mint leaves

- 2 quarts of water

Prep Time: 5 mins

Cooking Time: 0 mins

Total Time: 5 mins (plus chilling time)

Servings: 8

Nutrition Facts (per serving):

- Calories: 0

- Fat: 0g

- Saturated Fat: 0g

- Cholesterol: 0mg

- Sodium: 0mg

- Carbohydrate: 0g

- Protein: 0g

- Phosphorus: 0mg

- Potassium: 30mg

- Fiber: 0g

- Calcium: 0mg

Instructions:

1. In a large pitcher, combine the cucumber slices, mint leaves, and water.

2. Chill in the refrigerator for at least 2 hours, or overnight, to allow the flavors to infuse.

3. Serve cold, with additional cucumber slices and mint leaves for garnish.

Zucchini Bread Muffins

Ingredients:

- 1 1/2 cups whole wheat flour

- 1/2 teaspoon baking soda

- 1/2 teaspoon baking powder

- 1/2 teaspoon salt

- 1 teaspoon cinnamon

- 1/4 cup unsweetened applesauce

- 1/4 cup honey or maple syrup

- 1 egg

- 1 teaspoon vanilla extract

- 1 cup grated zucchini (water squeezed out)

- 1/4 cup chopped walnuts (optional)

Prep Time: 15 mins

Cooking Time: 20 mins

Total Time: 35 mins

Servings: 12 muffins

Nutrition Facts (per muffin):

- Calories: 100

- Fat: 2g

- Saturated Fat: 0.2g

- Cholesterol: 15mg

- Sodium: 150mg

- Carbohydrate: 18g

- Protein: 3g

- Phosphorus: 40mg

- Potassium: 95mg

- Fiber: 2g

- Calcium: 20mg

Instructions:

1. Preheat oven to 350°F (175°C). Line a muffin tin with paper liners or lightly grease.

2. In a bowl, mix flour, baking soda, baking powder, salt, and cinnamon.

3. In another bowl, whisk together applesauce, honey, egg, and vanilla. Stir in grated zucchini.

4. Add the wet ingredients to the dry ingredients, stirring just until combined. Fold in walnuts if using.

5. Divide batter among muffin cups and bake for 20 minutes, or until a toothpick inserted into the center comes out clean.

6. Let cool in the pan for 5 minutes, then transfer to a wire rack to cool completely.

Peach Sorbet

Ingredients:

- 4 cups frozen peaches
- 1/4 cup honey or maple syrup
- 1/2 cup water
- 1 tablespoon lemon juice

Prep Time: 10 mins

Cooking Time: 0 mins

Total Time: 10 mins (plus freezing time)

Servings: 4

Nutrition Facts (per serving):

- Calories: 120

- Fat: 0g

- Saturated Fat: 0g

- Cholesterol: 0mg

- Sodium: 0mg

- Carbohydrate: 31g

- Protein: 1g

- Phosphorus: 20mg

- Potassium: 285mg

- Fiber: 2g

- Calcium: 10mg

Instructions:

1. In a blender or food processor, combine frozen peaches, honey, water, and lemon juice. Blend until smooth.

2. Transfer the mixture to a freezer-safe container and freeze until solid, about 4 hours.

3. Before serving, let the sorbet sit at room temperature for a few minutes to soften slightly.

Carrot Cake Bites

Ingredients:

- 1 cup grated carrots

- 1 cup dates, pitted

- 1/2 cup oats

- 1/2 teaspoon cinnamon

- 1/4 teaspoon nutmeg

- 1/4 cup shredded unsweetened coconut

Prep Time: 15 mins

Cooking Time: 0 mins

Total Time: 15 mins

Servings: 12 bites

Nutrition Facts (per bite):

- Calories: 80

- Fat: 1.5g

- Saturated Fat: 1g

- Cholesterol: 0mg

- Sodium: 20mg

- Carbohydrate: 16g

- Protein: 1g

- Phosphorus: 20mg

- Potassium: 150mg

- Fiber: 2g

- Calcium: 20mg

Instructions:

1. In a food processor, combine grated carrots, dates, oats, cinnamon, and nutmeg. Process until the mixture comes together and forms a dough.

2. Roll the mixture into 1-inch balls. Roll each ball in shredded coconut to coat.

3. Store in an airtight container in the refrigerator until ready to serve. Enjoy as a sweet, nutritious snack or dessert.

14-DAY MEAL PLAN

Day 1

- ***Breakfast:*** Low-Potassium Apple Cinnamon Oatmeal

- ***Lunch:*** Tuna and White Bean Salad

- ***Dinner:*** Lemon Herb Baked Cod with a side of Grilled Vegetable Platter

Day 2

- ***Breakfast:*** Kidney-Friendly Egg Muffins

- ***Lunch:*** Chicken and Avocado Wrap

- ***Dinner:*** Vegetable Stir-Fry with Tofu

Day 3

- ***Breakfast:*** Berry Smoothie Bowl

- ***Lunch:*** Quinoa Veggie Salad

- ***Dinner:*** Quinoa Stuffed Bell Peppers

Day 4

- ***Breakfast:*** Avocado Toast with Poached Egg

- ***Lunch:*** Broccoli and Almond Soup

- ***Dinner:*** Baked Garlic Parmesan Chicken served with Cauliflower Rice Stir-Fry

Day 5

- *Breakfast:* Quinoa Breakfast Porridge

- *Lunch:* Mediterranean Lentil Salad

- *Dinner:* Herb-roasted turkey Breast with a side of roasted vegetables (from the Grilled Vegetable Platter recipe)

Day 6

- *Breakfast:* Spinach and Mushroom Egg White Omelette

- *Lunch:* Roasted Vegetable Quiche

- *Dinner:* Lemon Dill Salmon Pasta

Day 7

- *Breakfast:* Banana Walnut Pancakes

- *Lunch:* Turkey and Cranberry Sandwich

- *Dinner:* Balsamic Glazed Chicken with a side salad (lettuce, cherry tomatoes, cucumber, with lemon juice and olive oil dressing)

Day 8

- *Breakfast:* Almond Butter and Blueberry Smoothie

- *Lunch:* Grilled Chicken Caesar Salad

- *Dinner:* Spinach and Feta Stuffed Salmon with steamed green beans

Day 9

- *Breakfast:* Pear and Cottage Cheese Toast

- *Lunch:* Baked Salmon with Dill Yogurt Sauce served with a cucumber salad

- *Dinner:* Cauliflower Rice Stir-Fry

Day 10

- *Breakfast:* Carrot and Ginger Soup (served warm for breakfast for a comforting start)

- *Lunch:* Quinoa Stuffed Bell Peppers

- *Dinner:* Lemon Herb Baked Cod served with a side of roasted asparagus

Day 11

- *Breakfast:* Banana Walnut Pancakes

- *Lunch:* Vegetable Stir-Fry with Tofu

- *Dinner:* Balsamic Glazed Chicken served with a side of mashed cauliflower

Day 12

- *Breakfast:* Kidney-Friendly Egg Muffins

- *Lunch:* Mediterranean Lentil Salad

- *Dinner:* Grilled Vegetable Platter with Herb-Roasted Turkey Breast

Day 13

- *Breakfast:* Quinoa Breakfast Porridge

- *Lunch:* Turkey and Cranberry Sandwich

- *Dinner:* Lemon Dill Salmon Pasta

Day 14

- *Breakfast:* Berry Smoothie Bowl

- *Lunch:* Broccoli and Almond Soup

- *Dinner:* Baked Garlic Parmesan Chicken with a side of sautéed spinach

CONCLUSION

In conclusion, managing stage 3 kidney disease through diet requires careful consideration of nutrient intake, including the management of protein, potassium, phosphorus, and sodium levels, alongside adequate hydration. The comprehensive meal plans and recipes provided offer a balanced approach to eating that does not compromise on flavor or nutritional value, catering specifically to the needs of seniors with stage 3 kidney disease. From hearty breakfast options and nutritious lunches to satisfying dinners and delightful snacks and desserts, each recipe has been designed to support kidney health while ensuring dietary variety and enjoyment.

The importance of diet in managing kidney disease cannot be overstated. By incorporating kidney-friendly meals into their daily routine, individuals can play a crucial role in managing their condition, potentially slowing disease progression and improving their overall quality of life. The recipes provided not only adhere to the dietary guidelines necessary for kidney health but also embrace the joy of eating through flavorful and diverse culinary options.

Individuals managing kidney disease need to consult with healthcare providers or dietitians to tailor these meal plans and recipes to their specific nutritional needs and health goals. Adjustments may be necessary based on individual health status, dietary restrictions, and preferences to ensure that the diet remains balanced, enjoyable, and supportive of kidney health.

In crafting this collection of recipes and meal plans, the goal has been to demonstrate that a kidney-friendly diet can be both nutritious and enjoyable. By making informed food choices, individuals with stage 3 kidney disease can enjoy a wide range of delicious meals that contribute to their health and well-being. This approach to dietary management empowers individuals to take an active role in their health care, offering a positive and flavorful way to support kidney function and overall health.

www.ingramcontent.com/pod-product-compliance
Lightning Source LLC
Chambersburg PA
CBHW050816250726
48653CB00006B/2255